TWO-THIRDS OF UK MEN ARE OV

EAT. DRINK. DON'T DIET.

The Basics	4
Enjoy Eating	6
Carbs	8
Fruit and Veg	12
Processed Food	15
Meat	17

Fats	20
Bread	22
Gut Health	24
Take-Aways and Snacks	27
Food and Sex	30
Booze	36
15 Foods For Men	36

3

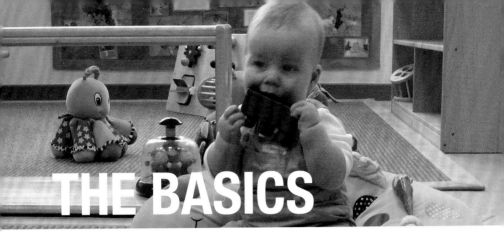

THE BASICS

There are thousands of diet books which is incredible because eating and drinking are actually pretty simple. It boils down (did you see what we did there?) to two things: energy and nutrition.

WHAT IS ENERGY?

The amount of energy in an item of food or drink is measured in **calories**. For most men, most of the time about 2,500 calories will give us more than enough energy to get through the day. Keep taking in more energy than you use and you'll put on weight.

In the UK, the average adult takes on 200 to 300 more calories every day than they need: the main reason why two-thirds of men are overweight or obese.

AND NUTRITION?

As well as calories, foods contain nutrients. All living things need these to survive and thrive. Humans need a variety of them.

The seven main classes of nutrients are **carbohydrates**, **proteins**, **fats**, **vitamins**, **minerals**, **fibre** and **water**.

We need more of some nutrients than others. To get them, we need to eat a variety of foods.

Starchy foods such as potatoes, bread, rice and pasta are our main source of carbohydrates (carbs). Choosing the whole grain (brown) version of these means you also get vitamins, minerals and fibre.

Beans, pulses, fish, eggs and meat are our main sources of protein.

Fruit and vegetables are major sources of vitamins, minerals and fibre which is why we're encouraged to eat five portions a day.

IS THAT IT?

Pretty much. Most foods contain more than one type of nutrient and in varying amounts. Food labels will help you see how much (or how little) of each nutrient you're eating. How they're prepared or cooked will make a difference too.

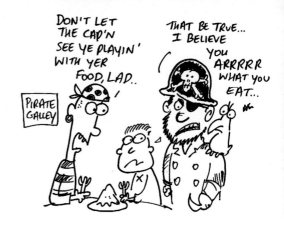

Calories you take on from foods or drinks without a lot of nutritional benefit - sugar, white bread, fizzy soda etc - are sometimes called 'empty calories'. You want to keep these to a minimum.

The rest of this booklet goes into more detail on the different types of nutrients and answers the most common questions.

WHY DO YOU SAY 'EAT, DRINK, DON'T DIET'?

If you want to eat more healthily (and even if you want to lose weight), diets with a capital D are not your best bet.

Diets involving meal replacements, faddy dishes or eating routines usually start well enough but they don't tend to last and rarely solve the problem. In fact, many dieters finish off carrying more fat than when they started.

Yo-yo dieting – where body weight repeatedly rises and falls – can be particularly unhealthy. Losing weight very quickly can actually result in lean tissue being lost rather than fat. Having less lean tissue can reduce your energy needs going forward and encourage weight gain.

Diets appear to help at first simply because they force you to think about what you're eating, but they don't last. The thing is they don't deal with the underlying problem: our attitude to food. Diets that 'forbid' foods and set up 'rules' and 'targets' turn food from a pleasure to a source of shame. Not a healthy feeling at all.

WHATEVER YOU DO, KEEP ACTIVE

Whatever you eat and drink, keep as active as possible. Every little helps. Aim for 10,000 steps a day - 15,000 steps if you want to lose weight. A pedometer (or a fitness monitoring device or app) can help.

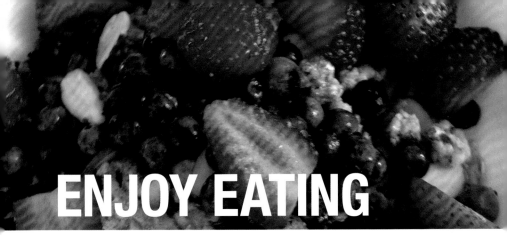

ENJOY EATING

You'll seldom meet a French person who is on a diet. No coincidence the French also top the league table for time spent eating and drinking. They enjoy two hours 13 minutes a day at their favourite activity. Bottom of the table is the USA - just an hour a day spent eating and drinking. In the UK, it's an hour and 19 minutes. (The international average is about an hour and a half.)

In France, the evening meal is often the centre-piece of the evening. Of course, the French snack but they don't blitz it. Why would you spoil the highlight of the day?

It seems counter-intuitive. But seeing eating as an important thing in life, something that is fun, an experience to be shared, to be savoured and to spend time on may actually mean you eat better.

Surveys of attitudes to spending suggest that many of us prioritise experiences over things. If that sounds like you, apply it to eating. Rather than seeing foods as things to be eaten, think of meals as experiences to be enjoyed.

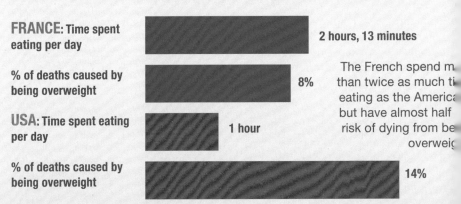

ENJOYING EATING MAY EVEN SAVE LIVES...

FRANCE: Time spent eating per day	2 hours, 13 minutes
% of deaths caused by being overweight	8%
USA: Time spent eating per day	1 hour
% of deaths caused by being overweight	14%

The French spend m than twice as much ti eating as the America but have almost half risk of dying from be overweig

HOW DO I DO THAT?

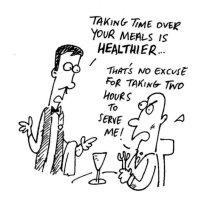

TAKING TIME OVER YOUR MEALS IS HEALTHIER...

THAT'S NO EXCUSE FOR TAKING TWO HOURS TO SERVE ME!

To start, don't even think about what you eat. Think about how you eat. Don't shovel it down in front of the telly.

Slow down. Look at your food. Chew it. Savour the flavour. Drink some water. You'll enjoy your food more and your body will know that it's actually eating. This is vital because it takes your brain a good 20 minutes to wise up that your stomach is full. This means that if you've been stuffing yourself, you'll have eaten more than you wanted.

An experiment compared chewing a mouthful of pizza 15 times before swallowing with chewing 40 times. The men who chewed 40 times were less hungry three hours later and had healthier blood sugar levels. Simple.

If you're struggling to slow down, try chop-sticks, smaller utensils or holding your fork in your non-dominant hand. Or spice it up: you might find you eat spicy food more slowly while the capsaicin in chillis and peppers may help your body's metabolism.

Once you're eating more slowly you'll taste your food better and enjoy it more.

THE ONE 'DIET' THAT DOES WORK

If you think you need the rules and discipline of a 'diet', try this one. (We can't really call it a diet because it doesn't ask you to change anything.)

> Prepare and cook your food in the same way and same quantity as usual.

> Serve only half.

> Put the rest in the freezer compartment for another time.

You get all your usual nutrients, just fewer calories. If you feel your plate looks empty, use a smaller plate. (Yes, it's that simple.)

If you can do it, it works. Halving your evening meal will see you losing about two pounds a week. Drink a glass of water ten minutes before you eat to take the edge off your appetite.

Most of us don't want to waste food. It's better for the planet and better for the wallet. So rather than bin or scoff what's left after a meal, why not freeze it or bung it in the fridge for another meal? Save calories, save cooking. Sounds obvious but it's amazing how we don't think of it.

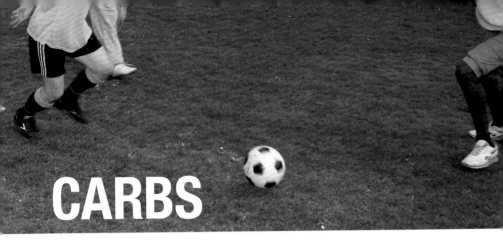

CARBS

Carbs are a main source of energy (and so of calories) but they aren't all the same. They contain different amounts of sugars, starch and fibre. These affect the speed at which carbs release their energy. This is measured using the glycaemic index (GI).

Foods that release energy rapidly and increase blood sugar have a high GI; foods that release their energy more steadily have a low GI. Generally the more sugar in a food, the higher its GI.

High GI foods trigger the release of insulin which pushes sugar from your blood stream into your body's cells. This insulin activity can lead to a fall in blood sugar shortly afterwards, leaving you feeling tired and struggling to concentrate.

HIGH GI > GO EASY

Parsnips, baked potatoes, cornflakes, raisins, donuts, bread, mashed potatoes, dried fruit.

MEDIUM GI > EAT MODERATELY

White rice, honey, boiled new potatoes, fresh apricots, bananas, potato chips, sweetcorn, porridge oats, muesli.

LOW GI > EAT MORE FREELY (BUT DON'T GO MAD!)

Carrots, lettuce, tomato, cucumber, peppers, small portion brown rice, mango, Kiwi fruit, unsweetened bran cereal, peas, grapes, sweet potato, baked beans, small portion wholewheat pasta (cooked al dente), orange, apple, pears.

A high GI lunch is the reason for that afternoon slump after eating, something that becomes more noticeable as you age.

Combining small amounts of high GI foods with those of lower GI helps prevent blood sugar swings.

It'll help your relationships too. Hunger related to low blood sugar levels is a major cause of domestic arguments (low blood sugar triggers anger because glucose is the major fuel for brain cells).

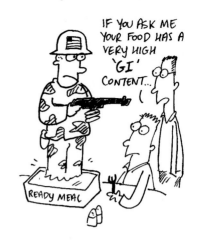

IF YOU ASK ME YOUR FOOD HAS A VERY HIGH 'GI' CONTENT...

READY MEAL

DO I EAT TOO MUCH SUGAR?

The health impact of sugar in our diet has become so clear over the last decade that in 2015, Public Health England halved its guidelines on sugar. The maximum recommended amount of so-called free sugars is now equal to about seven cubes of sugar (30g) a day. So don't add sugar if you can help it, and check food labels for added sugars and those found naturally in honey, syrups and fruit juice (even unsweetened).

If you think about all the sugar added to bread, cereals, biscuits, ready-meals, cakes, drinks, fizzy drinks and all the other processed food we eat, you get to seven sugar cubes quite quickly.

Look for the 'Carbohydrates (of which sugars)' figure on the label. Remember that even food marked low sugar can contain up to 5g of sugars per 100g.

Sugar can also be found hidden in the list of ingredients. Corn syrup and any ingredients ending in -ose are all sugars. Examples include sucrose, glucose, and fructose. Probably best avoided if they're near the top of the ingredient list.

No need to count the sugars found naturally in whole fruit and vegetables (and in milk and milk products like plain yoghurt). They're OK in moderation.

AN ORANGE IS OK BUT ORANGE JUICE ISN'T?

The sugar behaves differently. In a whole fruit (or dried fruit) the sugar is still within the fruit. The juicing process changes this. You could say it frees the sugars up. As a result they're absorbed into the body in much the same way as a spoonful of sugar, the unhealthy way.

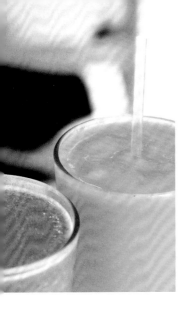

The easiest way to avoid the confusion is to choose whole fruit over shop-bought juices or smoothies.

Or make your own smoothie, perhaps including some veg to reduce the sugar content.

IS SUGAR ADDICTIVE?

Carbohydrates trigger the release of feel-good brain chemicals such as serotonin. This can make you crave similar foods. But, these effects are not as addictive as, for example, nicotine or alcohol. Ignore the craving for something sweet after a meal and it will pass.

Scientists have also found stress hormone receptors within the taste buds that detect sweetness which may explain why we turn to sweet foods when stressed.

If you crave something sweet, distract yourself. Exercise will do this best - a walk or run - as it will burn off the effects of stress and also curb the cravings - but anything that keeps you absorbed will help. If you can't get away, drink water or herbal tea.

CHOOSE LOW-SUGAR ALTERNATIVES?

Choose naturally low sugar products rather than those that use artificial sweeteners.

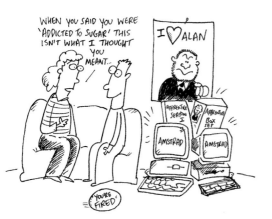

It may seem obvious to choose the diet version of your favourite soda - same sweet taste, no sugar. But if anything the sugary sensation in your mouth is even stronger than with real sugar which may increase cravings.

Some say it even tricks your body into thinking that since it is consuming a lot of sugar, it should lay some down as fat.

Certainly, diet soda drinkers appear more likely to be overweight and more at risk of diabetes.

SALT

Try to avoid eating more than about a teaspoon of salt a day in total (6g). Too much can raise your blood pressure, tripling your risk of heart disease or stroke.

That doesn't mean you can sprinkle a whole spoonful on your chips. About three-quarters of the salt we eat every day is already in the food, so try to avoid adding any salt at all if you can.

On food labels, check out the amount of sodium per 100 g. (You'll remember from your science lessons that the chemical name of salt is sodium chloride.) Over 1.5 g of sodium per 100 g is a lot and best avoided. Aim for 0.3 g maximum or 'no added salt'.

The red, amber and green traffic-light flashes on food labels can help you. As with traffic lights on the road, red means stop and green means proceed with caution. Obviously, you want as much green as possible.

Herbs and spices are a great alternative to salt to add flavour to food.

HOW TO READ FOOD LABELS

Most pre-packed foods have these traffic-light nutrition labels on the packaging which tells you how much energy, protein, carbohydrate and fat they contain (per 100g and often per serving, too).

In general, the more green on the label, the healthier it's likely to be.

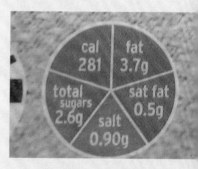

Ingredients are listed in order of quantity. If sugar is near the top of the list, it may contain more than is good for you. Similarly, if there are a lot of E numbers and words that sound more like chemicals than foods, you may want to steer clear.

Red on the label means the product is high in fat, saturated fat, salt or sugars.

> **22.5g of total sugars (per 100g) is A LOT**

> **1.5g of salt (per 100g) is A LOT** (0.3g is a little)

> **17.5g of fat (per 100g is A LOT** (3g is a little)

> **5g of saturated fat (per 100g) is a A LOT** (1.5g is a little)

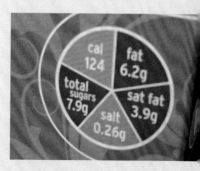

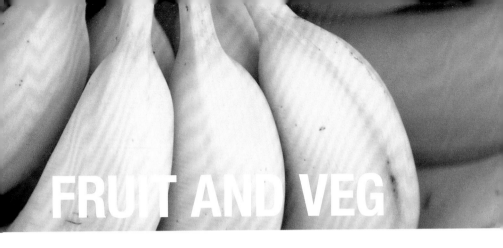

FRUIT AND VEG

The one thing we all know about eating is that we should try to eat five portions of fruit and veg a day. They're a great source of vitamins and minerals including vitamin C and potassium, and of dietary fibre. Hitting the 'five a day' target can help to lower your risk of heart disease, stroke and some cancers.

If you choose whatever's in season locally, you'll get variety throughout the year and help the environment by reducing food miles.

BUT WHAT IS A PORTION?

A portion is:

> part of a bigger fruit or vegetable (eg half a grapefruit or avocado),

> one medium sized piece of fruit or veg (like a banana or corn on the cob),

> two smaller ones (like two kiwis or heads of broccoli)

> three tablespoons of something cooked, canned or frozen

> a glass of fruit juice or vegetable juice (no more than one a day)

> a bowl of salad

Get a good mix of colours.

I DON'T LIKE VEG.

You probably do. The problem is often over-cooking.

Try them lightly steamed, stir-fried or flashed on a barbecue. Try more exotic options. Heard of rainbow chard, butternut squash or romanesco?

Buy what's in season - much cheaper and, if local, often fresher and tastier.

Sweet potato is an alternative to regular white potato - they're packed full of vitamin A - while vegetarian curries, Chinese and Thai meals are so tasty you won't miss the meat.

IS SOYA 'BAD' FOR MEN?

Soya (or 'soy' in the USA) is a great source of plant-based protein and nutrients. It may help lower cholesterol. But because it contains compounds that are similar to the female hormone oestrogen, questions have been asked about the impact of soya on the male hormone testosterone. The research suggests this is a myth: it makes no difference. Eating soya won't reduce your testosterone levels. In fact, it may even protect a little against prostate cancer.

There is, however, a good reason to go easy on the soy sauce: it's not the soya beans, it's the high salt content. (If you can, choose naturally fermented soy sauce; the cheaper chemically-fermented one may contain toxic compounds called chloropropanols.)

HOW CAN I EAT MORE VEG?

If you're having trouble eating five portions of fruit and veg a day, replace one serving of cereals, bread, pasta or rice with one of vegetables.

Learn the soup trick. It's an easy, tasty way to eat more vegetables.

A soup starter is less common in the UK than it once was. Not so in China where it's still the popular choice. It's great for portion control. Instead of wolfing down your main course because you're starving, a soup beforehand means you'll make better choices, eat more slowly and probably eat less.

Soup can also be a main course. A lot of us eat three times a day: breakfast, one big meal and one smaller one. The smaller meal is often a sandwich or something else that's easy to prepare (or buy at work). As the main part of this second meal, soup is ideal. It's not unusual in France, for example, to have soup in the evening if you've had your main meal at lunch.

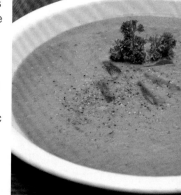

You can make a big soup and then eat it over several days. Fresh, frozen or tinned vegetables - whatever you fancy, they'll all do. Hack all the fresh veg up small (carrots are good to include). In your saucepan, fry chopped onion in a little oil or butter. Add a bit of garlic if you like (it doesn't have to be fresh, buy paste). Add boiling water from the kettle and chuck in all the fresh vegetables. A little salt and pepper. Some herbs. Let the fresh stuff cook a little then add any frozen and then any tinned veg (a tin of tomatoes is a good choice). Let it all cook through nicely. Use a blender to whizz it all up and add some milk. Soya or almond milks are good as they're creamier.

Fancy croutons? Just lob in some cubes of stale bread, no frying or toasting needed.

A vegetable smoothie works too. Carrots and beetroot are good choices and add some leaves of spinach or kale. You won't taste them. Add a bit of fruit for sweetness.

WHAT ARE ANTIOXIDANTS?

A lot of cell damage in our bodies which can lead to cancer is caused by unstable atoms, molecules or ions called free radicals. Antioxidants, which are found in many fruit and veg, can cancel out the cell-damaging effects of free radicals by binding with them.

Antioxidants include vitamins C and E, selenium, and carotenoids, such as beta-carotene and lycopene. (See the Favourite Foods For Men box on page 34 for some good sources.)

Lifestyle factors which can encourage the development of free radicals include fried foods, alcohol, tobacco smoke, pesticides and air pollutants.

SHOULD I TAKE SUPPLEMENTS?

For most non-vegetarian men most of the time, the answer is probably no. It's best to get all your nutrients from your diet if possible.

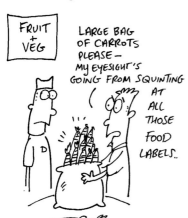

The one exception to this is perhaps vitamin D. Vitamin D, which is vital to bone health, is found in a few foods (oily fish, red meat, liver and egg yolks) and is also added to some food including fat spreads and cereals but not, in the UK, dairy milk.

However, the main source of vitamin D is sunlight and the NHS reckon that most of us in the UK don't get enough between October and early March.

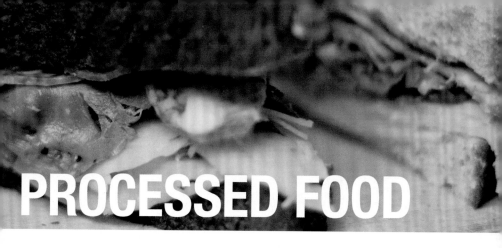

PROCESSED FOOD

A lot of our food is processed. Processed food simply means food that has been altered during preparation by, for example, freezing, canning, drying or baking.

There's nothing in principle wrong with it. It's handy and easy to use. But the more processing your food has been through, the more likely it is to have lost nutrients and gained sugars, salt and fats.

Baked beans are a good example of the problem. The beans themselves are very good for you but in the tins we buy they're often pumped up with salt and sugar.

WHAT CAN I DO?

Check the labels on tinned and other processed foods. You'll be surprised how much salt, sugar and other stuff is added. Try to choose the versions with the least salt and sugar.

Ready meals and convenience pre-packed options often have hidden salts and sugar too. So instead of a chicken meal, you could buy a chicken.

To make home-cooked meals more convenient, batch-cook and freeze extra portions for when time is tight. This means you get a home-cooked meal quicker than a take-away, cheaper and with more of the good stuff.

SHOULD I JUST BUY FRESH FOOD?

Generally the fresher the food, the more nutritious it is. But not all fresh food is all that fresh. Some will have been flown from the other side of the world. Fish tinned at sea or veg frozen when picked may well have more nutrients than an ageing platter packaged on the deli section to look nice and fresh.

Check out the country of origin of fruit and veg and buy local if you can.

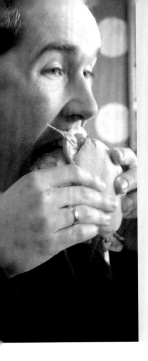

THE ENERGY DENSITY TRAP

Apart from the reduction in nutrients, some processed foods – and fast foods like burgers and fries too – have a high energy density. That means that each mouthful contains a lot of calories – more calories than your body is expecting. Human beings have evolved over thousands of years to guess how much we need to eat by the size of a portion, but just an ordinary looking portion of a high-density food can contain double the calories your body expects. If you also have the habit of putting it away like a wolf in a meat factory, you can see how the calories can mount very quickly.

Moreover, you can become dependent on the sweet, salty, fatty tastes because they give you an instant hit. In tests, rats that are used to this sort of food get the shakes when they're deprived of it.

SO, IS THE WAY WE EAT TODAY UNNATURAL?

The foods we eat now are very different from those we've eaten in the past. Humans like us have been on Earth for at least 200,000 years and 'homo' (human) species very similar to us for at least two million years. So relatively speaking, the cultivation of crops only began yesterday and the processing of food an hour ago.

For most of our time on this planet, we have been eating what we could hunt and what we could gather from the landscape around us. That means a diet of mainly fruit, nuts, vegetables and meat.

Not that the meat would be much like today's factory-farmed meat. Lean meat, free range, organic or game is closer to what we evolved eating.

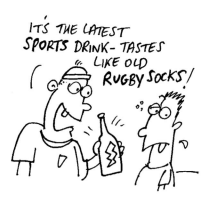

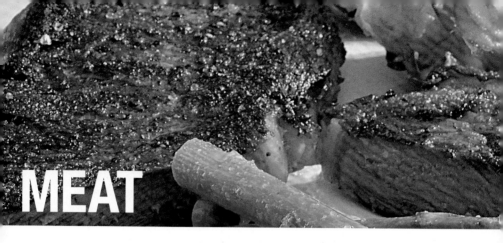

MEAT

The World Health Organization classifies red meat and processed meat as cancer-causing.

That doesn't mean they're as dangerous as tobacco or asbestos but it does mean you need to keep a close eye on how much you're eating.

It's hard to quantify the risk exactly but the NHS advises no more than 70g a day of red and processed meat. That's not a lot. The NHS reckons that a cooked breakfast containing two typical British sausages and two rashers of bacon is equivalent to 130g.

Red meat includes beef, lamb, pork and similar meats (not chicken, turkey or game).

Processed meat includes sausages, bacon, ham and deli meats.

Of the two, processed meat carries the higher risk - the World Cancer Research Fund advises eating 'little, if any, processed meat'. Also avoid heavily char-grilled meat (yes, that frazzled black stuff on your mate's barbecue!)

Having said all that, meat contains protein, iron, zinc, vitamin B12 and other nutrients that we all need to include in our diet.

Health-wise, there's not much difference between a low-meat and no-meat diet. However, most people do not become vegan or vegetarian for health reasons. There has long been concern about animal welfare. In the drive for more and more, cheaper and cheaper meat, it is the animals that suffer.

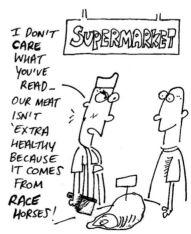

I DON'T CARE WHAT YOU'VE READ - OUR MEAT ISN'T 'EXTRA HEALTHY BECAUSE IT COMES FROM RACE HORSES!

SUPERMARKET

Recently, an arguably even bigger concern has emerged: the devastating impact on the environment and climate of livestock farming. Meat provides about 18% of human calories but uses 80% of the world's farmland while even the most environmentally-friendly beef products produce six times the global emissions of the equivalent plant protein. Meat production has snowballed to four or five times the level it was in the 1960s.

As the world's population continues to grow, the current model is unsustainable.

WHAT ABOUT PROTEIN IF I DON'T EAT MEAT?

There are many alternative sources of protein including fish, lentils, chickpeas, other beans and pulses, nuts and seeds, quinoa, quorn, mushrooms and cheese (especially cottage cheese which is lower in fat and contains more protein per calorie).

Broccoli and peas both contain protein. So do eggs and dairy products like milk and yoghurt.

Edamame beans are very trendy - they're baby soya beans.

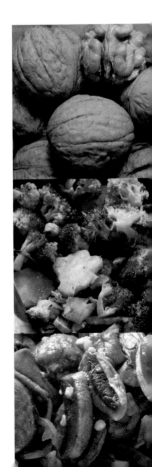

If you're cutting down on meat, you could try replacing half the meat in a dish with, for example, chopped fresh mushrooms - less meat but no loss of flavour.

WHAT ABOUT OTHER NUTRIENTS?

There are some nutrients that it is difficult to get without some meat in your diet. These include:

> Vitamin B12 which is important for brain function and energy is pretty much only found in animal-sourced food;

> Creatine and carnosine - important for muscles;

> DHA (docosahexaenoic acid) - important for the brain and mostly in fish; and

> Iron - although the iron in red meat is particularly well-absorbed by the body, there are many vegetarian alternatives including beans, pulses, nuts, seeds, grain and certain fruits and veg.

Supplements are available for most of these nutrients if you need them. Many vegans and vegetarians take B12, for example. Cereals and non-dairy milk can be fortified with B12.

On the positive side, a healthy vegan or vegetarian diet can reduce the risk of weight-gain, heart disease and some cancers. About one in eight Brits now say they are vegetarian or vegan with about a third of the population reducing their meat intake.

MEAT =

18%
of calories

80%
of farmland

BUT I LIKE EATING MEAT.

Meat substitutes are now everywhere.

Currently, the 'meat analogues', as food scientists apparently call them, include tofu (made from soya), tempeh (from fermented soya, like the kebabs below) and seitan (from wheat gluten) but the race now is to create the look and feel of meat: the 'blood', the fibrous texture.

The big food corporations are on board and the next few years will see meat analogues on plates across the world. These products should be far less environmentally-damaging than the meats they are designed to replace.

No doubt many of them will be very tasty but the thing to remember is that all these are highly processed foods with thickeners, emulsifiers, sugar and salt. 'Whole' foods they ain't.

The holy grail is to create meat from animal cells in the laboratory: real meat 'grown' without harming the environment or living animals. We have the technology to make this 'cultured meat' (or 'clean meat') but not yet at the price of a Big Mac.

When the world's first lab-grown burger appeared in 2013, it cost $330,000.

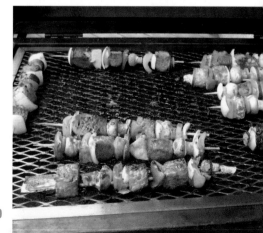

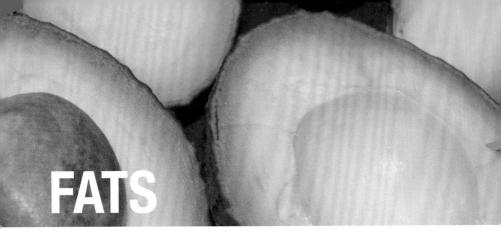

FATS

All fats are concentrated sources of energy (9 calories per gram compared to 4 calories per gram for carbs and protein) so go easy even on the healthy ones.

ARE THERE REALLY GOOD AND BAD FATS?

Monounsaturated fats (found, for example, in olive oil, nuts and avocados) and omega-3 fats (found, for example, in oily fish, rapeseed oil and walnuts) are called 'good' fats as they have beneficial effects on cholesterol balance in the body.

Some saturated (animal) fats are converted into cholesterol in the body which has seen them labelled 'bad'. But, as they are often present with good nutrients that minimise these effects, a little saturated fat is probably fine. For example, egg yolks are also rich in lecithin and vitamins.

The saturated fat in meat has been particularly demonised over the years but the real bad boys are not meat fats but trans fats.

WHAT ARE TRANS FATS?

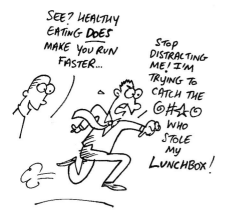

SEE? HEALTHY EATING DOES MAKE YOU RUN FASTER...

STOP DISTRACTING ME! I'M TRYING TO CATCH THE @#&@ WHO STOLE MY LUNCHBOX!

They're an industrial product created when vegetable oils are converted into something solid and 'spreadable'. They give foods a realistic feel in your mouth as well as a longer shelf-life.

It sounds harmless enough but worldwide, trans fats are responsible for half a million deaths a year according to the World Health Organization. In 2018, the EU adopted rules to eliminate them.

The UK food industry is trying to wean itself off trans fats. It is said they're not used in food processed here but that they are still found in food from abroad.

Look out for them in margarines, baked products, cereals, fried foods, sweets, chocolate products, spreads, soups, salad dressings, snacks, ice cream and frozen breaded products. There's no legal requirement to label trans fats specifically. Look for words like 'hydrogenated', 'shortening' and, of course, 'trans' on the food labels.

WHAT ARE ESSENTIAL FATTY ACIDS?

The fats in oily fish such as omega-3 are called essential fatty acids. They're essential because the body can't make them itself so we need to get them from our diet. Omega-3s are found in salmon, trout, mackerel, herring, sardines, pilchards, whitebait, tuna and anchovies.

Tinned fish is fine (and really easy to eat with pasta or pretty much anything). The tinned varieties of the fish above will, in general, with the exception of tuna, contain decent levels of healthy fats.

Shellfish like mussels, oysters, crab and squid also contain omega-3s. Shellfish are high in zinc too which helps male fertility.

White fish like cod, haddock, plaice and sea bass, while good for you because they're low in unhealthy fats, don't contain as many omega-3s. If you fancy some fish, choose it poached, baked or grilled rather than deep fried. Keep battered fish and chips as an occasional treat.

The NHS recommends at least two portions of fish a week, including one of oily fish. (However, don't eat more than four portions of oily fish a week as they can contain low levels of pollutants like mercury, especially from fish near the top of the food chain like swordfish or shark.)

As far as omega-3s in meat are concerned, grass-fed meat and dairy products are better choices than grain-fed ones.

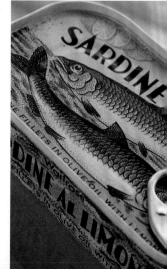

Omega-3s are also top of the list of nutrients for the brain. Neurotransmitters are the chemicals that carry signals between brain cells. Like all chemicals in the body, they can only be formed from the ingredients you make available – in other words, from what you eat.

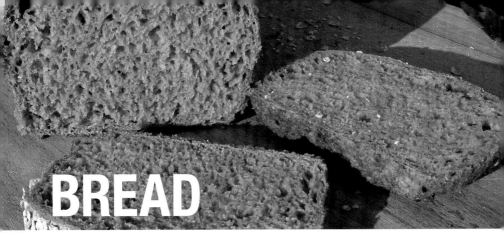

BREAD

Some breads are high in salt, some in fat, some in sugar, some in the lot. Often these loaves have healthy-looking images on the packaging. There is also a massive variation in calories with some breads having twice as many per slice as others. So check the labels on your favourite loaf.

The healthiest breads will be made from whole grains which retain all the natural nutrients including B vitamins, folic acid, iron, selenium, magnesium and fibre. Look for the word 'whole' on the ingredient list. If it ain't there, it ain't wholegrain regardless of how many healthy descriptions like 'multigrain' or '100% wheat' or 'unbleached flour' are plastered over the packaging.

Processed bread which is usually white removes the bran and germ from the wholegrain. It has a longer shelf-life and is easier to digest but has none of the good stuff: no fibre or vitamins and minerals. These are often added back in the manufacturing process but added vitamins and minerals are not as easily absorbed by your body as the real thing in real grains.

Too much white bread can increase the risk of diabetes, heart disease and obesity.

Even if you do find the word 'whole' on your ingredient list, look out for added preservatives, salt and sugar.

WHAT ABOUT GLUTEN?

Unless you have coeliac disease or a genuine gluten-intolerance, gluten is fine to eat. Avoid gluten for no good reason and you may find yourself missing out on whole grains. Research suggests that while eating gluten doesn't cause heart disease, avoiding whole grains so as to avoid gluten might. (Sourdough, fermented bread, is lower in gluten.)

Some people have an intolerance to wheat rather than gluten. If you think that bread or similar products are making you feel bloated or uncomfortable, get it checked out by a doctor rather than just assuming you're gluten-intolerant.

DO-IT-YOURSELF

Want to be sure of your bread?

Bake it yourself. It's fun. Slightly messy fun. You tend to get absorbed in what you're doing which makes it good for mental health. A bread-making machine can simplify it if you don't have the time or inclination but still fancy a bread you know to be fresh and full of nutrition.

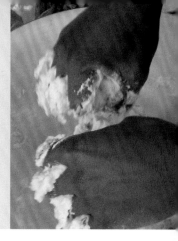

SHOULD I EAT BREAKFAST?

Having gone without fuel overnight, you need to fill the empty tank. If you don't, you may well eat more than you need later in the day because you're hungry, perhaps grabbing easy but less healthy snacks.

However, research suggesting that breakfast eaters are healthier than non-breakfasters probably says more about the people than about the meal. That is to say that, as a rule, people who eat breakfast probably eat more healthily generally than those who don't. So provided you eat well the rest of the time, skipping breakfast is of itself probably not bad for you.

For breakfast cereal, choose wholegrain versions such as shredded wheat, Weetabix, porridge or unsweetened muesli. (Granola is full of good stuff but high in calories.) And obviously, if you're having something else for breakfast, all the info in this manual still applies.

Want to cut down on sugar? Changing cereal could be the way. Check the label on yours.

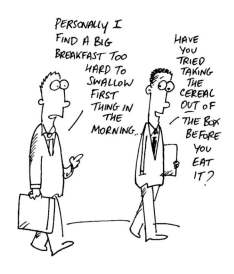

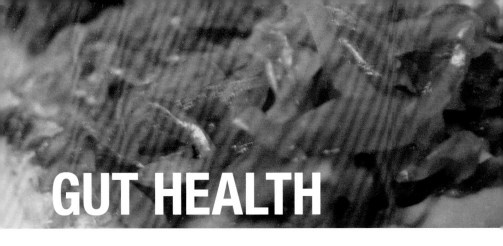

GUT HEALTH

Good health begins with a healthy gut - it helps everything from your heart and brain to your digestion, immune system and sleep.

In your gut, there are apparently more than 50 trillion microbes from over 1,000 different species. (Gulp.) As ever it's high fibre, whole foods, fruit and veg that you need to eat for good gut health. They help so-called good gut bacteria (probiotics) to thrive while antibiotics and processed foods do the opposite.

Bloating, diarrhoea, constipation, cramps and gas may all be signs of poor gut health. Irritable bowel syndrome (IBS) affects about 11% of men. Don't just rely on over-the-counter treatments. It's important to see your GP to check the cause is not something else like Crohn's disease, colitis or coeliac disease (caused by a gluten-intolerance).

People with IBS may need to avoid what are sometimes called fodmap foods. It stands for Fermentable Oligosaccharides, Disaccharides, Monosaccharides, and Polyols. Snappy.

Fodmap foods are basically various types of carbohydrate that are poorly absorbed by the body. Common offenders include onion, garlic, wheat and animal milks. If you think you might be affected, get some advice from a doctor or nutritionist.

Time can take its toll on our guts, especially if we've taken lots of antibiotics. Eating more slowly will help.

Don't take probiotic supplements without guidance from a health professional.

SHOULD I EAT FERMENTED FOOD?

Fermented foods are particularly rich in probiotics and will give your gut a helping hand. Common fermented foods include:

> Kefir (fermented milk)

> Sauerkraut (raw cabbage)

> Tempeh (soya beans, Indonesian)

> Natto (soya beans, Japanese)

> Some types of cheese (including cottage cheese and ricotta)

> Kombucha (tea)

> Miso (soya beans)

> Kimchi (cabbage and radish, Korean)

> Yogurt (fermented milk, fewer healthy bacteria and less protein than kefir)

> Sourdough bread

> Olives

Not all fermented products are friends of your gut. Salami (fermented meat, usually pork) and beer and wine should be consumed in moderation.

ARE MILK AND DAIRY OK?

Milk and dairy products like cheese and yoghurt form part of a healthy diet. They are great sources of protein, calcium and B vitamins - but go easy: they contain saturated fat. Try semi-skimmed or low-fat instead of full-fat.

For putting on cereal, skimmed milk is fine. Or try unsweetened, low-fat yoghurt/fromage frais or non-dairy milks such as soy, almond, coconut, rice or oat milks. Look for milk alternatives that are calcium-enriched. Add fresh berries, nuts or chopped fruit for extra flavour.

Some people are lactose-intolerant. They cannot digest milk because they don't produce enough of the enzyme, lactase, to process lactose sugar found in milk. Try the non-dairy milks mentioned above or goat's milk.

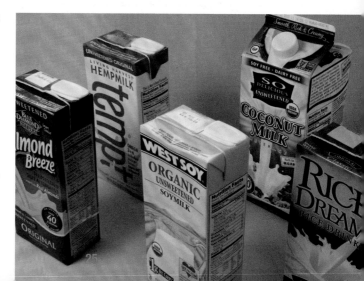

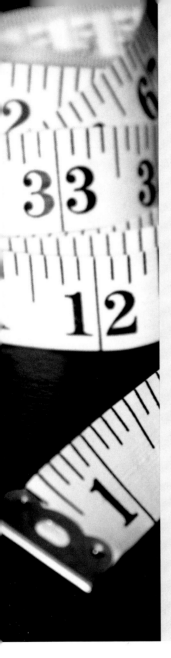

ARE YOU OVERWEIGHT?

Adult obesity has pretty much doubled since the early 1990s. Two-thirds of UK men are now overweight or obese, putting them at greater risk of a heart attack, heart disease and cancer.

The standard official measure of how heavy we should be in relation to our height is called the Body Mass Index (or BMI). You can work out BMI like this:

Weight (in kilograms) / height (in metres) squared

A healthy BMI is anything between 18.5 and 25. Anything below 18.5 is considered underweight. Over 25 is overweight and over 30 is classified as obese.

So generally if your BMI is over 25, you're overweight and need to act.

But it's complicated a bit by ethnicity. Asian men are advised to keep BMI even lower - below 23 - because of their increased risk of diabetes. Black men and some other minority groups are strongly advised to keep it below 25 for the same reason.

BMI can also be misleading because muscle is heavier than fat. This means that some sportsmen - rugby players, for example - can easily have a BMI that, on the face of it, looks too high.

MEASURE YOUR WAIST

It is easier just to measure your waist. That will give you a good enough guide. Your waist measurement is not your trouser size. Measure at the widest point, probably level of your belly button. If it's over 37 inches (94 cm), then you're probably overweight; if it's over 40 inches (102 cm) then you're probably obese.

CAN YOU WALK OFF A MEAL?

Light exercise after eating reduces the rise in blood sugar and fat levels that can increase the risk of weight gain, raised blood pressure and cholesterol and type 2 diabetes. Watch out for cramp or heartburn though.

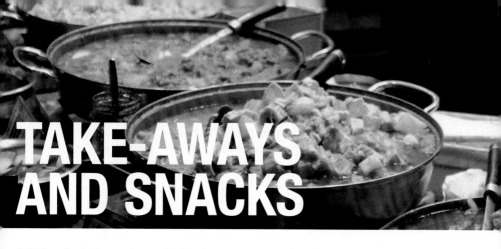

TAKE-AWAYS AND SNACKS

A little of what you fancy is fine but not every day. Balance a big meal out or takeaway feast with what you eat at home the rest of the week. The more you eat out, the more you need to be aware.

Know your menus. Did you know ghee (in Indian food) is clarified butter or that soy sauce is high in salt? Everybody likes to eat with a man who knows his way round a menu so learn more about cooking styles and ingredients and what the dishes really contain.

Some menus give calorie and health information. If you're after the healthier options, avoid foods wrapped in pastry or fried, deep-fried, battered foods or fritters and go for grilled, baked or steamed dishes instead. Look out for buttery or creamy sauces. And also watch chutneys and pickles - they're often full of sugar and salt.

Having a takeaway is a chance to try something different like a fish or a vegetarian option. Or a salad.

Don't go large. On the contrary, you could order less takeaway and do your own side of brown or wild rice and/or salad etc.

Sharing desserts and starters is fun and means you get to try more stuff. Healthier too.

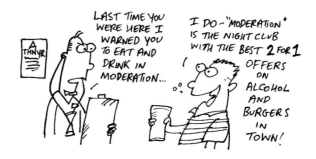

	Top choices...	Go easy on...
Indian	Tomato-based sauces or dry curries (rogan, jalfrezi, tandoori, bhuna), dhal (lentils), chana (chickpeas), saag (spinach so high in nutrients)	Creamy options (masala, pasanda, korma), bhajis, naan
Chinese/ south-east Asian	Steamed dishes, soups, chop suey (chicken), stir-fry (veg), summer roll (translucent rice paper covering)	Fried or battered dishes, crispy duck, sweet and sour, spare ribs, prawn crackers, too much soy sauce, spring roll
Italian	Thin crust, lean meats, tomato sauces, reduced-fat mozzarella	Deep pan or stuffed crusts, fried dishes (calamari), lasagne
Chippie/ burger bar	Plain grilled fish (breadcrumbs, maybe), mushy peas, thick cut, wedge-style chips, grilled chicken	Thin cut or triple-cooked chips, battered stuff, onion rings etc. (Watch out for soggy batter - suggests oil wasn't hot enough so more fat absorbed.)
Mexican	Fajitas, burritos (especially bean options)	Fried or refried dishes, salty chips, nachos, sour cream and cheese.
Kebab	Vegetable, shish or chicken	Doner

DRINK WATER

Some claim a health boost just from drinking more water. It's certainly the best fuel going. We function better when properly hydrated. Try a glass of water or tea instead of a snack.

Check your snack attack isn't due to thirst - drink enough fluids to keep your urine a pale straw colour, not dark yellow or brown.

A glass half an hour before a meal can also take the edge off your appetite.

I SNACK WHEN I FEEL DOWN.

Studies show we are more likely to eat junk when we're fed up but find it easier to make healthy choices when happy. It's a virtuous circle since if you eat healthily, you're more likely to feel good and cope better with stress.

The nutrients in healthy foods, and the feelings of enjoyable eating influence your mood: you make better decisions without realising. They also improve your sleep.

Since we're less likely to make healthy choices when hungry or stressed, beware when shopping after work (when you might be feeling both).

HOW CAN YOU BEAT A SNACK ATTACK?

Beat a snack attack with exercise (even gardening or housework will do it). It's worth it as just a few biscuits a day surplus to your calorie needs can see you put on half a stone in a year and add inches to your waist.

If you do succumb, a small carbohydrate snack (biscuits, pretzels etc) may only spike your blood sugar and leave you craving more carbs, try a protein snack (unsalted nuts, seeds, dried fruit, yoghurt, cheese, apple with a little peanut butter...).

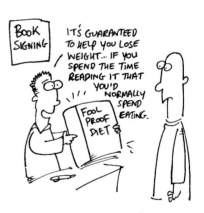

SNACK CHECK

Check labels. A snack is likely to represent a healthy option if, per 100g, it contains:

> less than **3g fat**

> less than **2g sugar**

> less than **0.25g salt**
    (or less than 0.1g sodium)

A snack is best avoided if, per 100g, it contains:

> **20g** or more **fat**

> **10g** or more **sugar**

> **1.25g** or more **salt**
    (or more than 0.5g sodium)

For snacks with values in-between, handle with care.

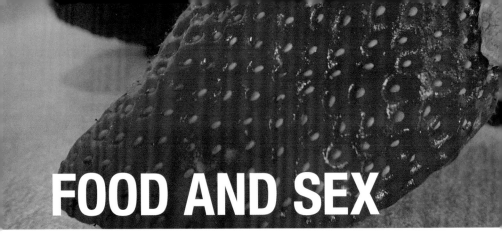

FOOD AND SEX

CAN I IMPROVE MY SEX LIFE BY CHANGING MY DIET?

Along with more sleep and more exercise, tweaking what you eat can make a difference to your sexual energy, testosterone levels, fertility and stamina.

Being overweight reduces the amount of testosterone available to the body so that's a good place to start.

Also address any vitamin or mineral deficiencies, especially in zinc and magnesium. Eat more seeds (particularly pumpkin and sunflower seeds), dark leafy greens, shellfish, beans, yoghurt, fish and lean meat. Sprinkle some nuts and seeds on your stir-fry.

Get your 5-a-day fruit and veg, regular weekly portions of seafood and a daily handful of unsalted seeds and nuts and you won't go far wrong.

But while diet will help, other changes will help your sex life far more.

WHAT OTHER CHANGES?

Exercising more, stopping smoking and keeping an eye on the booze.

Alcohol increases desire but can make erections poorer. With heavy, long-term drinking erectile dysfunction can become regular. Longer term, heavy boozing can also shrink your testicles and lower sperm count. (More on alcohol on page 32.)

CAN FOOD AFFECT YOUR SEX LIFE?

YEP- STOPPED MY GIRLFRIEND EATING CHIPS OFF MY PLATE. NOW I'M SLEEPING ON THE SOFA.

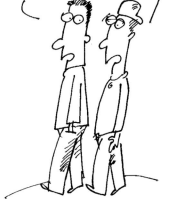

THE SEXIEST NUTRIENTS...

Sexual Function	Nutrients	Food sources
Healthy testosterone levels and sex drive	Vitamin A	Animal and fish livers, kidneys, eggs, milk, cheese, yoghurt, butter, oily fish, meat, margarine, dark green leafy vegetables and yellow-orange fruits
	Magnesium	Soya beans, nuts, yeast, wholegrains, brown rice, seafood, meat, eggs, dairy products, bananas, green leafy vegetables, dark chocolate, cocoa
	Zinc	Red meat (especially offal), seafood (especially oysters), yeast, wholegrains, pulses, eggs, cheese
Healthy Sperm	Vitamin C	All fruit and veg, especially citrus, blackcurrants, guavas, Kiwi fruit, peppers, strawberries, green sprouting vegetables
	Vitamin E	Oily fish, fortified margarine and dairy products, liver, eggs
	Selenium	Brazil nuts (the richest source), other tree nuts, broccoli, mushrooms, cabbage, radishes, onions, garlic, celery, wholegrains, yeast, seafood, offal
Stamina and staying power	B vitamins	Yeast extracts, brown rice, wholegrain bread and cereals, seafood, poultry and meat (especially offal), pulses, nuts, eggs, dairy products, green leafy vegetables
	Iron	Red meat (especially offal), seafood, wheatgerm, wholemeal bread, egg yolk, green vegetables, prunes and other dried fruit
	Iodine	Seafood, seaweed, iodised salt
Arousal and orgasm	Calcium	Milk, yoghurt, cheese, green vegetables, oranges, bread
	Phosphorus	Dairy products, yeast, soya beans, nuts, wholegrains, eggs, poultry, meat and fish

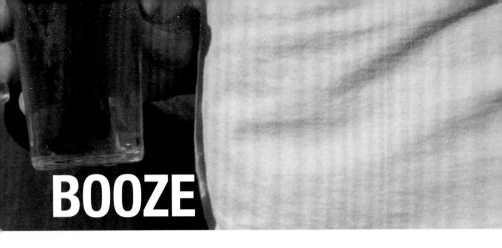

BOOZE

Alcohol is probably the most popular drug in the world. Like any other drug, if you're going to take it, you need to know how it works.

At its best, alcohol can be part of the fun of being with other people. At its worst it can kill. Second only to tobacco as a killer, alcohol is responsible for five times more deaths worldwide than all the illegal drugs put together.

Anyone at any time could develop a problem with alcohol, including you.

In the UK, the Chief Medical Officers say there is no absolutely safe level of drinking. They advise no more than 14 units a week including some alcohol-free days and to avoid binge drinking (more than six units in six hours).

WHAT DO YOU MEAN BY A UNIT?

A unit is eight to ten millilitres of alcohol, which is about two teaspoonfuls.

Drinks sold in bars may all be different sizes but in theory they have about one unit of alcohol in them. One unit = one 30 ml glass of spirit (a single measure) = one 100 ml glass of wine = half a pint of ordinary 3.5% beer. But it's not easy. A light Australian or American beer may be 3% alcohol or less. Many craft beers are twice that. Watch out for glass sizes too. Some large wine glasses are close to a third of a bottle. And then there are the cocktails...

Information on units of alcohol is not always user-friendly. Most bottles and tins carry some information from which you can – with a degree in advanced mathematics – work out how much alcohol you're actually drinking.

There's more on alcohol in the Forum's manual Serious Drinking.

For example, say you have a 33 cl (centilitre) can of beer, which contains five per cent alcohol. This 33 cl equals 330 ml (millilitre), so you multiply 330 by 0.05. This equals about 16. This means that there is 16 ml of alcohol in the can, which is about two units.

WHAT EFFECT DOES ALCOHOL HAVE?

Too much alcohol can cause high blood pressure and heart disease. It can cause stomach problems such as ulcers and cancers of the throat, mouth and tongue.

Alcohol is processed in the liver. Liver disease kills ten times as many heavy drinkers as non-drinkers and 80% of liver disease is caused by alcohol. In parts of the UK the number of people getting liver disease has doubled in the past ten years.

Alcohol is fattening. (It's made from sugar.) Alcohol is 7 calories per gram, compared to around 4 calories per gram for carbohydrates. A pint of beer contains about 185 calories – 30 calories more than a 28 g packet of crisps. It also makes you feel hungry. Put the two together and you get the beer belly or, to put it another way, fat in the most dangerous place for heart disease.

Alcohol can encourage risk-taking. In Europe, drunk drivers kill 10,000 people every year. That's more than one death per hour.

Alcohol is a factor in break-ins, muggings and sex offences. Offenders are under the influence of alcohol in the majority of violent crimes. Alcohol is also behind two out of five incidents of domestic violence.

Alcohol is a depressant. It is involved in as many as two out of three suicides. If you're drinking because you're unhappy, get support.

Any risk is increased if you mix alcohol with other drugs – legal or illegal. If you're on medication, check with your GP how much you can drink.

Find a soft drink you like (preferably something low-sugar). Making your first drink a soft one (or water) will help cut alcohol. It'll quench your thirst and rehydrate you too.

DO I HAVE A DRINK PROBLEM?

Some people with problems with alcohol are very good at hiding it from both others and themselves. If you're worried about yourself, then that alone should be warning enough to cut down and, if you can't cut down, to stop.

It's not your fault if you have no control over alcohol. It's just the way you are. But you do need to admit it. If the booze is boss, you need to stop. If you don't, alcohol will kill you.

An early warning sign that you might be at risk is if you get drunk very easily and/or have memory blackouts when you drink and can't remember what happened.

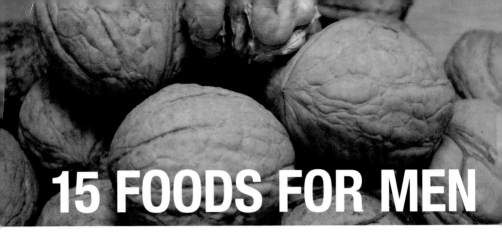

15 FOODS FOR MEN

There's no such thing as a superfood but these are all very good for men.

> **Broccoli** - betacarotene, omega-3s, vitamins C and E plus B vitamins, calcium, iron and zinc. Yes, there's no such thing as a superfood but broccoli comes pretty close.

> **Carrots** - the richest source of betacarotene (all orange and red veg are a good source, perhaps try sweet potato if you don't like carrots).

> **Citrus fruits and pineapple** - vitamin C (pineapple juice is not dissimilar to stomach acid so it's not great for your teeth).

> **Garlic** - a natural antibiotic – the king of healing foods is good for cholesterol and blood pressure. (For best results, eat fresh garlic as soon as possible after chopping but pastes are easier and pickled garlic a less smelly alternative.)

> **Ginger** - full of good stuff, ginger is a natural prevention for travel sickness and nausea. (By the way, both garlic and ginger are said to be good for your sex drive.)

> **Walnuts** - top non-animal source of omega-3 fatty acids and a great source of antioxidants. (Also high in antioxidants are pecans, chestnuts, peanuts and pistachios. Most nuts are good for you but beware of calories and added salt and sugar.)

> **Sunflower seeds** - top seed for antioxidants especially vitamin E (two tablespoons - 28 g - daily will double most people's vitamin E intake). Other antioxidising seeds include poppy seed, linseed, sesame seed and pine kernel. Pumpkin seeds are also high in zinc and magnesium and may be good for your prostate, sperm quality and sex drive.

> **Chilli** - high in vitamin C and betacarotene, chili also boosts calorie burning.

> **Tea** - high in antioxidants called flavonoids. Choose lighter tea (oolong, green, jasmine) for maximum benefits.